My Cane and I

A Memoir of a Disability

Tony Tripodi

iUniverse, Inc.
New York   Bloomington

My Cane and I
A Memoir of a Disability

iUniverse books may be ordered through booksellers or by contacting:

iUniverse
1663 Liberty Drive
Bloomington, IN 47403
www.iuniverse.com
1-800-Authors (1-800-288-4677)

Because of the dynamic nature of the Internet, any Web addresses or links contained in this book may have changed since publication and may no longer be valid.

ISBN: 978-1-4401-2878-3 (pbk)
ISBN: 978-1-4401-2880-6 (cloth)
ISBN: 978-1-4401-2879-0 (ebk)

Library of Congress Control Number: 2009924018

Printed in the United States of America

iUniverse rev. date: 3/6/2009

Preface

This book is a quasi-memoir about my use of a cane to manage leg and hip pain. It is a memoir in the sense that many of the events described are based on actual interactions with others. It is "quasi-" because it covers a very few years of my life, and some of the events are either distorted by my memory and perceptions, or are subjected to the product of my imagination. Real and imaginary perceptions are clearly delineated; and names of real persons described in the book are either omitted or disguised.

Part One deals with how I came to use a cane, and with personal experiences in learning about canes, pain management, and medication.

Part Two includes vignettes of different episodes I've experienced and imagined in my interactions with others. The descriptions are sometimes painful, sometimes fanciful, sometimes hilarious, sometimes tragi-comical.

Acknowledgements

I especially thank Dr. Karen Randolph for her support and encouragement to write this book. And, I am grateful to those people, unknown to me who exhibited their unsolicited kindness and concern in their interactions with those of us who use canes. Finally, I am grateful to Rachel Koechlein for typing the manuscript, and the editors of i Universe for preparing it for publication.

Contents

Why Do I Need A Cane?

I'm a retired professor from a large university in Ohio. Retired for three years, I discovered I had to use a cane to help me walk. The cane has become a part of me, an appendage. I rely on it to manage my leg and hip pains.

When I was a runner, regularly jogging and competing in road races, I adhered to the runner's creed: no pain, no gain. Many years later, my cane walker's slogan is less pain with a cane.

My story begins with how I came to realize I needed a cane. It is based on my perceptions and fantasies of cane users as well as those who have yet to experience adventures in the cane world.

I retired from academic administration, research, and teaching at the age of 72. When I tried to walk a straight line, I walked with a serious limp, swinging from side to side. Most certainly, I could not have passed a breathalyzer test; yet I wasn't drunk. One faculty person commented that I walked funny. Unlike Johnny Cash, I wasn't able to walk the line. My physician in Ohio told me I had arthritis, and the cartilage between the bones on my left leg and hip was gone. The hip bone wasn't exactly connected to the leg bone. It was bone against bone. I had little agility in my leg, and I was warned that I would probably need surgery.

Deathly afraid of hospitals and operations, I allowed the good doctor's advice to enter one ear, probably the left one, only to exit from the right ear on a direct line to outer space. I obviously could not walk the lines in either outer or inner space.

My thoughts of hospitals, operations, and doctors bordered on primitive thinking and illogical fears. Since I had an excellent education from two very prestigious universities, the University of California at Berkeley and Columbia University, one might have thought I should have been able to employ sound methods of logic in my daily endeavors. However, logical thinking for me existed only in the classroom.

Because I witnessed in two different hospitals the deaths of my mother and father, an irrepressible logic informed me that people die in hospitals. Therefore, causing Aristotle's bones to rattle in his grave, I thought I would die if I went to a hospital. Of course, my fuzzy brain dismissed the fact that I was born in a hospital and survived two other hospital stays. I even witnessed the birth of my children in hospitals; and indeed, they did live and are still alive.

I left Ohio without undergoing surgery. Still limping along without a cane, I moved to Boca Raton, Florida, where my wife lived. For eight years we had a commuting marriage, living together in the summer and visiting each other at least once a month during the rest of the year. It was intended that the commuting part of the marriage would end, and I would settle down happily in retirement. Suffice it to say, along with some physical pain, I felt the psychological pain of a deteriorating relationship.

Tired of my short, happy retirement life, I applied for visiting professorships in other parts of the country: the University of California at Berkeley for one half year, followed by another year at Hunter College in New York City. Fortunately or not, I received both professorships, and my odyssey to Berkeley and New York City began.

At Berkeley, after some marital counseling in Florida, it was clear that both the commuting and non-commuting aspects of the marriage were doomed. My ex and I filed for divorce and property settlement in Florida, and the marriage was dissolved between my time at Berkeley and at Hunter College.

While visiting Berkeley, the pains in my leg and hip continued to grow. Perhaps, my psychological pain from a failed marriage metastasized to my leg and hip? Despite the pain I did not think of using a cane, neither to manage physical pain, nor to deal with psychological pain. A magical cane might have come in handy at that time in my life. However, the only cane I experienced was candy cane during the Christmas holidays. It should have been sweet, but somehow it became bitter.

I was bitter because I had no health insurance. Previously I was covered by my wife's insurance policy. Just as she became an ex, so did my insurance coverage. It wasn't until I settled in at Hunter College that I was eligible for health benefits. Reluctantly I made an appointment with an orthopedic surgeon to obtain a diagnosis regarding my leg and hip. The pains had increased geometrically, and it was more difficult to walk.

Dr. OPERATE NOW was very efficient. He had x-rays taken and seemed to take great pleasure in giving me the bad news. I had severe arthritis. My left knee and hip were dysfunctional because there was no cartilage between the bones. This was similar to what the good doctor in Ohio told me previously. However, Dr. OPERATE NOW had more doom and gloom to report. He indicated my right leg would soon be dysfunctional and I needed an operation immediately! Dr. OPERATE NOW said he no longer operated. While he recommended the names of several available surgeons, I noticed that he limped. This, for some strange reason, reminded me of my visit to a young, obese cardiologist who prescribed lipitor to lower my bad cholesterol count. Within months of his recommendation, I was told he died, naturally of a heart attack. Could OPERATE NOW have had a hip operation?

Equipped with a packet of x-rays and the names of several surgeons eager to operate, I returned to my apartment in New York City. Apprised of the bad news, I was anxious and depressed. I felt that I had no one to take care of me after an operation, and I didn't know whether I could afford the cost of nursing care.

What to do? Like any normal American afraid of doctors and the health system, I decided to take control. I opted to obtain a second opinion. Maybe even a third and fourth opinion until hopefully I could hear what I wanted to hear, i.e. no operation.

A friend advised me to consult one of the top orthopedic specialists in New York City. The doctor was not included in my health plan; more than likely because he was too expensive. Nevertheless, I decided to seek his consultation. I showed Dr. OPERATE LATER the x-ray pictures taken by Dr. OPERATE NOW. The doctor briefly examined me and came to a quick decision. Eventually I would need surgery to replace my hip; however, I could wait. The purpose of the hip operation would be to reduce the pain. After an operation I would need six to 11 months of rehabilitation, and I would probably still limp. Dr. OPERATE LATER informed me I should use a cane if I didn't get an operation.

Why use a cane? Dr. OPERATE LATER said it would reduce 50 percent of the pressure on my leg, resulting in less pain. When (and if, I thought) I would be ready for an operation, I would know. What he meant was the pain would be so unbearable that I would want an operation. The logic for acquiring a cane was irrefutable. With no cane there would be a great deal of pain and no gain. With a cane there would be less pain. Ergo, it would be insane not to get a cane.

I was thankful for the advice of Dr. OPERATE LATER. The 10 minute consultation for $500 was well worth it because I was not ready to undergo an operation. Nevertheless, as prone as I was to illogic and to disobeying medical recommendations, I had to reflect on whether I could manage pain without an operation or a cane.

Can I Manage Pain?

I did some serious thinking about whether or not I should go ahead with an operation rather than postponing it, leaving my pain reduction to medication and a cane. This meant that I spent a couple of days talking to myself.

I'm not very logical when I think of life and death choices, particularly as they relate to me. The chief advantage of an operation, according to Dr. OPERATE LATER, was that my pain would be reduced dramatically. In contrast, Dr. OPERATE NOW thought I would find myself shriveled up and confined to a wheel chair and/or bed if I weren't operated on immediately. Incidentally, my relatives seemed to side with Dr. OPERATE NOW.

On the negative or disadvantageous side of the ledger regarding my life, I decided on these reasons for not wanting to have an operation:

1. I was afraid I would die under anesthesia. Basically, like Hamlet, I thought that I would sleep, even dream. But there's the rub. In that dream of sleep I would never wake up.

To investigate this further, my quasi-logical mind prompted me to think of what experiences I had under anesthesia. There were two. One occurred when I was hit by a car while jogging and had go into surgery. This was 21 years ago, when I was 55. Needless to say, it was not a very good year. I didn't die; however I was in a kind of drunken state for several days after the operation. My friends thought I acted strangely. Of course, I did not participate in the decision to operate. I was told it was necessary since I was close to dying.

The other experience wasn't exactly a planned use of anesthesia. It took place in Ohio when I was 65. I received a local anesthetic to dull the pain in my gums when they were scraped by an orthodontist. After the procedure I asked Dr. OXYCONTIN if I could drink a little sherry along with the oxycontin for reducing pain.

"No Problem," said Dr. OXYCONTIN.

That night I took oxycontin, the prescribed dose, and drank a little sherry. Soon after, I passed out in the bathroom. I fell to the floor, breaking the sink. An hour or so later, I awoke on the floor with a sore back and a broken sink.

I muttered to myself "I could have died. I'm not taking that stuff anymore."

Much to my chagrin, I also had to pay the landlord for a new sink.

So, I survived these pain killing experiences; and I escaped death both times. Now that I'm older I fear the possibility of a heart attack during an operation. I take lipitor, amlodopine-benaz, and baby aspirin daily; but who knows what will happen when anesthesia and these medicines interact. More than two thirds of operation failures might be attributed to procedural mistakes and/or physicians' errors for all I know.

2. If an operation should be successful, I fear what life would be like in my semi-mechanical state with an artificial hip.

I doubt I would yell, "Hip, Hip, Hooray." More than likely, I would utter, "Please hip, don't slip!"

Slip, slip, sliding away, I would be afraid there would be no one to help me. How could I cope alone? Would I be able to travel to Italy and other romantic places? Or would I, in this gas guzzling economy, think of shorter jaunts to more attainable places like Hells Kitchen, Mud Flats, or Salt Mines?

My very educated friends and relatives might say this about being afraid to have an operation; "There's nothing to fear, but fear itself, according to F.D.R."

I would be told I could obtain a visiting nurse while in rehabilitation. But I wasn't sure I could afford it. Nor did I relish the idea of paying for a nurse. I won't even pay for a housekeeper, preferring to clean my apartment in my own lackadaisical style. My bottom line was that I was afraid of confinement and possibly not being able to drive to places during a lengthy period of rehabilitation.

Having considered these reasons for not having an operation, I thought I should remain open to other possibilities. I knew I didn't want an operation, hoping to postpone it indefinitely; yet I searched literature, especially magazines and newspapers, for more information. The strangest bit of information I gleaned was some patients who had hip operations found themselves squeaking; i.e., there were squeaks in their artificial hips. I imagined myself like the tin man in the Wizard of Oz, needing oil or some other lubricant to keep me going. Perhaps, I would carry a can of WD40 and spray my hip from time to time.

I began to manage hip pain in Ohio by taking Aleve and Tylenol. Aleve seemed to work better but it had the disturbing side effect of raising my blood pressure. However, my physician thought it was all right to use Aleve because I only had a mild case of hypertension. I also tried Ben Gay and Icy Hot. The odors bothered me, and those analgesics didn't appear to work well. I tried Ben Gay with a vanishing scent, discovering the scent only vanished slightly and the pain didn't vanish at all. It was just as effective to use no medication and simply rub my hip with my hands.

When I ran in road races, I used to rub Ben Gay and/or Icy Hot on my legs. A burning sensation was created, and it made me feel that my legs were limber rather than a few degrees separated from rigor mortis. Unfortunately, these balms had less of an effect as I aged and arthritis invaded my body.

To ease my psychological and bodily pains in Berkeley, I took to drinking very cheap, dry, and sweet sherry. The pains didn't subside, but I mistakenly believed the alcohol would help me feel better.

I noticed that my bodily pains were temporarily reduced when I felt angry. That might have been due to an adrenalin rush, surfacing as a distraction to pain. Again, my illogical brain emerged. I thought if I could induce pain in other parts of my body, I could reduce the pain in my hip. Nice try! It didn't work! I ended up with twice as much pain, but in different parts of my body.

Back in New York City after consulting with Dr. OPERATE LATER, I decided to explore the possible uses of a cane. Nevertheless, I continued to hope there was a magical cure (not an operation!) to reduce my pain.

I prayed to statues of Mary, Jesus, and St. Anthony at St. Patrick's church. The statues did not answer my prayers. Maybe my pain was a punishment from God or from one of her/his representatives. Receiving no help from my religious icons, I thought I would try some kind of alternative treatment such as acupuncture and acupressure.

An Adventure With Acupuncture.

From My New Jersey apartment I see an old man with ivory white hair walking on the boardwalk. His head and shoulders are stooped and he's walking at a very brisk pace. Like a metronome, he taps the boardwalk with his cane, step by step. I wonder if I'm looking at a projection of my image, but then I notice his cane is white with a red end. It isn't I. I'm not blind. As I hear the tap, tap, tapping of his cane, I think back to my first use of a cane in New York City.

I began to use a cane in daily walks to Hunter College. I soon realized that Dr. OPERATE LATER said nothing about the possibility I might develop blisters on my cane hand. Well, I did! However, the additional pain soon diminished. The blisters healed, and I officially became a calloused cane man.

One day at Hunter College, I struck up a conversation with a faculty person who noticed my limp. Professor PAIN SPOTTER told me he had pains which were relieved by acupuncture and he suggested I give it a shot. Seeking an alternative for pain reduction, I jumped at the chance (Not really! I wasn't able to jump at all. But you get the picture. I became excited!). Professor PAIN SPOTTER recommended Dr. WOO, an acupuncturist who was gentle, knowledgeable, and helpful. The professor thought it was worth a try, suggesting it might reduce pain and increase my ability to walk the line. He undoubtedly noticed when I limped, I veered from left to right (or was it right to left?).

I made an appointment with Dr. WOO the next day. I indicated I probably needed an operation but I was hoping to find some relief. She described a treatment plan of five sessions. Along with a fear of anesthesia, I was also squeamish about shots and needles. My history with needles was one of utter fear and distaste. Whenever blood was taken from me in a physical examination, I had to look away. As an example of my vulnerability, many years ago I gave blood to my mother; and the result of that was I fainted.

Sensitive to my concerns, Dr. WOO began to woo me. She indicated her needles were very thin, and I would hardly feel them. Cowardly as I might have seemed, I thought I was on the frontier of a new courage. To most people, it would have been a trifling experience. To me, it was like being on the edge of another world. Dr. WOO and I discussed the costs of treatment which unfortunately were not covered by my insurance. I decided to go ahead anyway. In the words of professor PAIN SPOTTER, I thought it was worth a try.

The following week I kept my first appointment. Dr. WOO's office was above a store that sold herbs, tea, and other exotic Asian surprises. I hoped I could buy fortune cookies and General Tso's chicken. No such luck!

I expected to have a fortune that read, "Today is your last day of pain."

It wasn't in the cards or in the cookies. I suppose that's the way the cookie crumbles; or in other words of an articulate society, it is what it is!

To arrive at Dr. WOO's office I had to climb a long, steep stairway. At the top was a receptionist who escorted me to a dark room where I was to undress and put on a smock. That I did. Dr. WOO soon began the treatment. I told her, perhaps looking for sympathy, I was like a baby when it came to needles. She said she'd be gentle, and there would be little pain.

I was truly in a mysterious world. Lying down with my face buried in a pillow, my legs and hips were punctured with needles. Although it was more painful in my imagination than in the flesh, I felt that my body was in a purgatory infested with flaming needles. Dr. WOO turned off the lights and told me to rest for one half an hour. It was eerie, kind of spooky.

When Dr. WOO returned to remove the needles, I felt a burden lifted from my body. I was relieved of real or imagined pain from the needles. Dr. WOO then proceeded to rub me in spots identified as pressure points.

At the end of the treatment session, she helped me with my clothes, hugged me, and asked if I felt better. Being of a sound academic mind, I couldn't say yes or no.

I spoke my kind of truth: "I feel better since the needles were removed. However, I still feel the pain in my hip, and I'm tired."

Dr. WOO smiled and assisted me down the stairs. She optimistically indicated I would feel less pain in the next session.

The next session I lay on my back, and the needles were inserted on the front of my legs. Again, I didn't look at the needles. I shut my eyes, only opening them when the treatment was finished. I felt exhausted and somewhat depressed. Energy was drained from my body. So much so that I cried. And then I became embarrassed. Dr. WOO kissed my forehead and hugged me until I stopped crying. She helped me down the stairs at the end of the session.

I thought, concurring with Dr. OPERATE NOW, my hip was too far gone. There was no cartilage to serve as a cushion between bones.

Nevertheless, I decided to finish the treatment. There were three more sessions.

Disturbed by the fact that my energy was sapped and I cried, I consulted with a friend who had experienced acupuncture. He told me that he had similar feelings after one of his treatment sessions. That made me feel a little better about my reaction to acupuncture.

I endured all five of the treatment sessions with no diminution in my leg and hip pains. Dr. WOO suggested that I needed something more basic than acupuncture. I needed a WOMAN, someone to love. She might have been right, but I didn't want to discuss it.

Dr. WOO said she had a perfect woman for me. "How about it?" she asked.

"I don't think so," I responded.

Dr. WOO, possibly an expert in the ancient art of wooing, told me to think about it further. That evening I received a call from her asking if I wanted the woman she selected.

I said, "No!"

After that call I immediately made plans to change my phone number (which I was in the process of changing anyway). Rather than wooing me, Dr. WOO's efforts shooed me away. For all practical purposes my adventure with acupuncture convinced me to pay more attention to my cane and less to alternative treatment.

I needed to learn more about my cane and how it could help me. I definitely wanted to explore the practice of using a cane in greater detail. So, what is a cane anyway?

What Is A Cane?

As a retired academic, I couldn't simply say a cane is a stick that helps one to walk. First, I had to define my terms, and then amass available information. I began my search about canes and their significance by using the internet.

I googled the word cane, and I discovered that CANE refers to the Classical Association of New England. It is an organization that has annual meetings, a summer institute, a president, and an executive committee. I instinctively knew that was not the right cane for me. I could hardly imagine consulting an executive committee every time I wished to take a step.

Back to google! This time I discovered an entry from Wikipedia, the free encyclopedia. The reference was retrieved from http:// en.wikipedia.org/wiki/cane. So what I'm about to write may appear to have some authenticity. The first thing that I learned is that a cane is a wooden stick, and can be made from different kinds of wood such as bamboo, rattan, or other plants.

More informatively, I learned that walking sticks were used in ancient times; not only to aid in walking, but also to be used to repel thieves and animals. I must have known this; for I carried a stick with me when in my youth I worked one summer as an engineering assistant for the U.S. Geological Survey. I used the stick to ward off scorpions and snakes in a Nevadan desert.

Canes were once a part of a gentleman's wardrobe in the 18th century. Evidently, the cane replaced the sword as an accessory to a gentleman's attire. I imagine I'm less likely to be arrested nowadays if I sport a cane rather than a sword. On the other hand, I'm sure the sword would be more useful to repel stray dogs.

It is interesting that a cane in earlier times seemed to symbolize the trappings of the upper classes including executives, rulers, and the like. However, that doesn't seem to be true today.

Wikipedia even referred to collectors of canes who gathered novel, interesting, and, perhaps, bizarre types. For example, some cane collectors obtained canes made from the penises of bison or bulls.

Canes can be used in many different ways. A James Bond type of person into action events might have within the hollow of a cane a sword. That would enable a gentleman to cut across the centuries using his cane as a walking stick and a sword. The cane hollow might even contain a vial of alcohol, an iPod, a sound recording system, and/or a camera.

Like Teddy Roosevelt or a leader of a Massai tribe, I could carry a big stick. A smaller stick with a hook shape at the end of it (like my cane) would not be as impressive because it would represent the need for power rather than power itself. Obviously, I am relegated to a little stick.

As a result of google explorations, I discovered a variety of fashionable and expensive canes. This information might have been helpful when I purchased my first cane. However, I might have been influenced to spend much more money.

Surfing the web, I discovered very distinctive canes made from woods like ebony and blackthorn. They were crafted from cane making experts from other countries. These are a few of the sub-categories of canes: anatomically correct, colortone classics/inlaid woods, derby handle, royal walking canes, and so forth (retrieved from http://en. wikipedia.org/wiki/cane). One sub-category that caught my attention was the Irish Blackthorn/Shillelagh. It was touted as useful against rabid people or animals that may be roaming in one's neighborhood.

I thought there must be other meanings of the word cane. Paying homage to my Italian American heritage, I noticed that CANE in Italian is a word for dog. Is using a cane like having a dog on a leash? Probably not. On second thought, however, a blind man who has a white cane with a red bottom might symbolically use his cane as a seeing eye dog. When one uses a cane to ward off animals, the cane can be thought of as functioning like a dog. I know canes can strike, although they don't necessarily bite. One might even put a sign on his cane, CAVEAT CANIS, beware of the dog.

In my search to uncover the meaning of cane, I thought (erroneously as it turned out) the significance of a cane could be enhanced by thinking of words that rhyme with it. A person who is caned can either be beaten or intoxicated. And, raising cain (notice this refers to the biblical older brother who murdered his sibling, perhaps because he was more able) refers to getting in trouble or having a good time, depending on one's predilection for pain or gain.

I compiled a list of rhyming words such as attain, bane, deign, feign, gain, lane, main, pain, quatrain, reign, seine, vein, wane, and so forth. This exercise wasn't very useful unless I wanted to be an ad man, pitching words to sell canes. The cane that mainly reigns over pain can be your gain for only thirty dollars. Or, the canes in Spain are mainly on the plains.

To complete my quest for the meaning of cane, I employed my academic skills. I consulted a dictionary. The only one I had was

Compact Oxford English Dictionary of Current English, Third Edition, Edited by Catherine Soanes and Sara Hawker, Oxford University Press, 2005.

Cane was defined in these ways:

"1. The hollow jointed stem of tall reeds, grasses, etc., especially bamboo.

2. The slender flexible stem of plants such as rattan.

3. A woody stem of a raspberry or related plant

4. A length of cane or a stick used as a support for plants, a walking stick, or for hitting someone as a punishment."

Basically, I learned from my search that a cane is a plant and/or a stick that can be used in many different ways. The stick is made of wood, but can also be made of metal as a substitute for wood. These generalizations don't depict what my cane means to me; nor do they begin to describe what a cane symbolizes to thousands of people who use canes.

My cane represents many different feelings as I have learned to accept and use it to cope with pain. I recognize that it's not the physical dimensions and characteristics of a stick that matter to others. Rather, it is their subjective interpretation of me as a cane user.

What do people observe when they encounter cane users? What is it like when one first uses a cane?

On First Using A Cane

I knew I had to start somewhere in my new cane world. Of course, I needed to acquire a cane. I looked on the internet and noticed very beautiful and expensive canes. However, I didn't trust my ability to successfully order a cane. That became clear to me when I once tried to order a gift from the internet and discovered I made six orders instead of one. It required several weeks of discussion with the company and my credit card bank to correct the mistake. Besides, diverting attention from my computer ineptitude, I thought the canes were too costly. I wasn't looking for a gold trimmed cane that would impress the people I, as an imaginary gentleman, would supposedly greet. As a result of my miserliness, I resorted to an old fashioned method. I walked to a Walgreen's drug store and looked for an inexpensive cane.

No canes were available. I went to another drugstore and arrived at the same conclusion. Subsequently I asked a pharmacist. She said there was a Walgreen's pharmacy that sold canes about a mile away. So I limped along for another mile, entered the store, and asked where the canes were. At least, the sales person didn't answer in a New Yorker, smart a—kind of way. He didn't say they're out walking, in Miami at the Orange Bowl, or in the Florida Everglades.

"Over there," he said, pointing at a cane made of dark brown wood with a hooked handle.

The cane cost ten dollars, a good buy! With my newly acquired knowledge gleaned from the internet, I wondered whether the darkened cane was an old plant or, in my wildest imagination, if it were a fossilized penis from some old bull.

As I started to walk with the cane, I thought of a bull goring some unlucky toreador while grunting, "Ole!" I too shouted "OLE" when I discovered I could successfully hold the cane in my right hand, tapping the ground in synchrony with my left foot.

To keep from slipping I had to be careful when I pressed the cane down on the sidewalk. Whenever the cane slipped, I slipped. Perhaps, it was a cane law of cause and effect. Nevertheless, I finally got the hang of cane walking.

My most embarrassing episode of cane management occurred when the streets of New York were icy and covered with snow. I manipulated my cane so that it was on top of a sewer cover. The cane slipped, and I slipped and fell. Naturally, I landed on my sore leg and hip. Fortunately, I didn't break any bones. Good Samaritan like New Yorkers picked me up without losing a step as they hurried to catch a bus. They told me I stepped on a sewer cover which was more slippery than the streets and sidewalks. Armed with that information, I walked slower, taking shorter steps, seeking to avoid sewer covers.

Although I felt uncomfortable, I was getting used to cane walking. I did feel less pain when I used the cane. However, I felt 10 years older and that people were watching me slip, slip, sliding away. I was self-conscious, but the equal opportunity New Yorkers treated me like anyone else walking on crowded streets in wintry weather. They pushed, shoved, and bumped to reach their destinations as quickly as possible.

It was not easy for a cane walker to use public transportation in New York City. I didn't ride on the subway because it involved walking up and down stairs, which was painful.

Traveling by bus for Italian lessons at the Berlitz School in Rockefeller Center was memorable. When I got on the bus I apologized to the driver for being slow, particularly as others were clamoring to be seated. The driver was also in a hurry. He was primarily interested in whether I had the right change.

Standing on the bus, I used my cane as a tripod, which was fitting since my last name is Tripodi. My cane as a third leg helped me to achieve some balance. However, it was difficult to stand; for the goal of the bus driver seemed to be to jerk, stop, and start, time after time, thereby tossing passengers from side to side.

New Yorkers who coveted their seats averted looking at me while I was standing. The hale, hardy, and young kept their seats, while the old and frail offered them. I guess it made the old and frail feel more youthful, hale, and hardy than I. In turn, I refused offers of the old and frail, so I could feel more youthful, hale, and hardy than they.

Bus drivers were on a mission to go as fast as they could and to be as unfriendly as possible. A story in the newspaper about an older, disabled person who was hit by a bus warned me to take time in crossing streets.

It was not easy for me to get off a bus. I had to hop down the steps and be prepared to land upright. Drivers, of course, had no worries about slowing down. Rarely would a bus driver be helpful in preparing passengers for a stop. Asking questions often led to a smart New York response, which usually resulted in missing my stop by one to three city blocks.

To hail a taxi was taxing. In my healthier days when I didn't have a cane, I could outrun other prospective passengers. With my newly found slowness, however, I missed many taxis. One night after the opera I spent two hours trying to hail a cab. I wound up walking and catching a bus to arrive at my apartment.

When I lifted my arm up with my cane pointed skywards and yelling, "Taxi", others crowded in front of me. They demonstrated that it was a jungle out there. Only the fittest survived the Taxi struggles.

The most successful strategy I employed was to stand by a hotel entrance, wait for a taxi to pull up, and then race for the taxi door. This didn't always work because others were able to barge their way into the taxi before I could.

Driving my own car was manageable, but still complicated. I lived on the Upper East Side in New York City where it would have cost $750 per month to keep my car in a garage. It was too much of a hassle to try to find a parking space on the streets every day, so I parked my car in a garage in Queens for $190 per month.

I had no difficulty driving, but it was painful to situate my self in the driver's seat. It was even more painful to ride in the passenger's seat, for I had to bend myself in awkward positions to fasten the seat belt.

Riding as a passenger in my son's car was like a carnival ride. He loved driving his BMW with a sports driving package; and he was very careful not to dirty his car with smudge spots. One day he barely waited for me to fasten my safety belt as he roared off. Showing his skill at zigging and zagging at high speeds, he seemed to be showing off or trying to make me sick. I tried to get him to slow down by asking why he needed to race his car. That had no effect. Then, I had a bright idea (the light bulb in my head was flashing). I told him that if he didn't slow down, I would have to vomit, thereby soiling his car. It worked! He slowed down, and my nausea subsided.

Shopping was a chore for a cane walker. I had to use one hand to manipulate my cane, push elevator buttons, and open doors. The other hand was used to carry groceries in plastic bags with handles. My problem was that I tended to carry too many bags, thereby straining my left shoulder.

Shopping was easier after I moved from New York to New Jersey, where I could comfortably drive to a supermarket. I'd park the car, get a cart, shop, load up the car, and use another cart, if available for bringing the groceries to my apartment.

I didn't escape New York drivers entirely. This was due to the fact that shoppers, who also drove in New York, pushed shopping carts the same way they drove their cars. Elderly people pushed their carts slowly, oblivious to others. While talking on their mobile phones, young people pushed their carts as if they were racing cars. The task for shoppers was to shop without getting hit by other carts and to finish in a reasonable amount of time without waiting behind some person who was day dreaming or a young housewife who was yelling at her children while chatting with two or three desperate housewives.

After shopping one day I thought I lost my cane. I immediately noticed the extra pain when I began to walk. I drove back to the store where I shopped and located my cane still lying in the cart I used for shopping. Fortunately I recovered the cane. Yet I began to think of it as an appendage, knowing that it was also necessary for me to take medication to reduce the pain in my leg and hip.

Pain Medication

I learned that the use of a cane could relieve some pain, but I quickly realized medication is also necessary. As I grew older and arthritis infested my body, I increased my drug intake. Below the age of 60 I took no medication on a daily basis; and I jogged, walked, and exercised. I believed I was in good health. I rarely visited doctors and had very few physical examinations.

In my 60's I used medication more frequently as I experienced more pain. A visit to a cardiologist indicated I had high cholesterol counts that could not be controlled by diet and exercise. Dr. HEARTBEAT, the cardiologist, prescribed Zocor and then Lipitor to render my good and bad cholesterol counts within normal ranges.

Dr. HEARTBEAT was relatively young and obese. As a warning that mortality is inevitable, he died from a heart attack. Could there have been more irony in my health care? Paradoxically, I distrusted doctors for physical examinations and surgery, but I relied on them for advice on medication. It was alright to hear them talk, but I didn't want them to touch me.

I tried to control hypertension with diet and exercise, but I was unsuccessful. I could no longer exercise vigorously and I increased my intake of Tylenol and Aleve. Unfortunately, a side effect of Aleve was that it was related to increased blood pressure.

Entering my 70's, I received medication for high blood pressure. Amlodopine-benaz was responsible for lowering my blood pressure to normal readings, even while taking Aleve. So this is now my daily medication: Lipitor, Amlodopine-benaz, baby aspirin, and Aleve or Tylenol.

I believe that medication is often a life saver especially for those with heart conditions. Drugs can reduce pain, but over reliance on them for every possible malady (colds, flu, fever, etc.) may not be helpful. Addiction to pain killers and other drugs can be lethal. At least, that's what my reading of magazines and newspapers indicates.

When I see others with their canes, I have no idea of the pain they must endure. Nor do I know the extent to which they take medication. Nevertheless, I wonder about their health as I do mine; and I think about the degree to which canes can assist in diminishing pain. But for a short period of time, I had a strange reaction to my cane. I wondered whether the cane was a bane on my life.

The Bane Of My Cane

My cane became part of me. Unlike my left leg, it was functional. It assisted me in walking and was something to learn on when I was standing. Yet, I began to resent the cane. Resentment at my not being as mobile and agile as I was in my younger years was displaced to my cane. It was as if the cane created my disability. It was illogical, but I continued to act as if it were the case. In other words, the cane became my bane.

It was the cane that made it difficult to shop; one hand for the cane, the other for carrying groceries.

It was the cane that led me to refuse seats offered on the bus. And, it was the cane that made me resent those offers. Obviously, I was ambivalent about people helping me. I really wanted to be taken care of, to be more comfortable sitting rather than standing on a fast moving, jerky bus.

Often when help was offered, I felt like throwing my cane away and walking off into the sunset (or was it the wilderness?). I was reminded of a time when I started to receive skiing instructions. After struggling to put on all the equipment (boots, skis, etc.), I was ready to learn how to ski. The instructor didn't think so. In a crisp, Teutonic accent, he yelled, "Turn left."

I fell down. He said in an even sterner accent, "You fell down."

I thought to myself, "No s---!"

The scenario was repeated over and over with the instructor's criticisms of the obvious ringing in my ears. I wished I could have got up, said something nasty, and skied away. That didn't happen. I simply said, "That's enough for today."

I never returned for ski instructions. As a reminder of my stubbornness, I sometimes fantasize about discarding my cane, exhibiting grace and agility in walking away.

There was a time in Italy when my daydream was partially realized. I didn't have a cane, but I was limping quite badly. I was late for catching a ferry boat to Sardinia. Instinctively, I ran. I must have generated a great deal of adrenalin; for I ran quickly. Arriving at the ship, I returned to my reality, limp, limp, limping along.

From time to time I would dream I was running and enjoying it. I felt the rush of euphoria after running many miles. However, while dreaming, I told myself, "This is a dream. I'm not really running. I have to accept it. I have a bad leg and hip."

I knew there was no gain in my terrain without a cane. Yet, I continued to regard the cane as my bane. Realizing that it was my body and not the cane that caused me to limp and be in pain, I was somewhat depressed as is evident in a poem I wrote: The Loss of Hope.

I know poems are not necessarily perceived as helpful. To me, they are a mode of expressing inner feelings. Whenever I suggested to a friend or relative they might be interested in reading one of my poems, their eyes swirled around, looking askance. It was as if I were some kind of pervert. More simply, they might have regarded the poetry as second rate. Or they might not have been really interested in my inner feelings.

The Loss Of Hope.

The storm raged
over white capped waves,
as my emotions were
tossed about
in a dizzying pace.
High waves swirled in rhythm
with Van Gogh's Starry Night
whirling in shades of cobalt blue
and deep ocean jade.
I stared at the distant horizon
where hope lived
in great beauty
for a brief moment in time.
Echoes of hope reverberated
in my brain,
vanishing in dark eddies
of despair,
sinking to the bottom
of the sea, somewhere.
1. From <u>Love and Hope by the Sea</u>, Tony Tripodi
     i Universe Press, New York, 2008.

The Cane Mutiny

I thought of my cane in two different ways: as a useful device to help me walk and as the bane of my life. I was ambivalent about using it. In contrast, in my imagination, the cane, anthropomorphically speaking, was ambivalent towards me. It took pleasure in assisting me, but disliked my constant bitching.

Every other day I walked by the ocean without a cane. Erroneously I believed that would help to strengthen my dysfunctional leg. In my walks I limped along the boardwalk for a mile or so, watching the seagulls, wishing I too could fly. That was a wish I developed when I saw my first movie. Judy Garland in The Wizard of Oz sang Somewhere Over the Rainbow, wondering why she couldn't fly over the rainbow like birds can.

It was obvious I had difficulty walking, let alone impossibly flying. When I was a boy, I donned a cape and jumped off a garage roof, hoping I could fly like superman. At night I also dreamt I jumped and subsequently floated in the sky for a long period of time. Sigmond Freud and Erica Jong who had a fear of flying would have regarded such a dream as the sexual yearnings of a young boy.

On the days I walked without a cane, my cane rested. If it were human, it would have been relieved to have a respite from my wimpy like ambivalence. At one point the cane was actually alive in the plant world, but in its state as my cane it wasn't even a shadow of its former self.

While walking near my apartment one day, a young woman said, "Where is your cane?"

I was somewhat in a daze and responded, "I probably left it at home."

When I returned to my apartment, I noticed the cane was gone. I might have left it at a restaurant or at a store, but I couldn't find it. Perhaps it was a cane mutiny in which the cane managed to lose me, or was it my mutiny in which I unconsciously lost the cane? It was a ten dollar stick, the color of dark mud. It helped me reduce some pain but caused my hand to blister.

What occurred to me was that people, like the young woman who noticed I didn't have my cane, are aware of and really notice others. I had become a fixture on the Pier Village scene, limping with my cane in hand. It was then that I thought it would be helpful to write about my perceptions of cane experiences as well as the perceptions others have of those of us who walk with canes.

In a perverse manner, rather than taking the cane mutiny as an omen of despair, I regarded it as a sign of hope. I would buy a new cane and I would write about my cane experiences.

Within a few days after the loss of my first cane, I was hoping to hear a band concert across the street from my apartment. However, it was cancelled due to a heavy rain. The rain soon stopped, and magically a double rainbow appeared over a wide expanse of the sea. It was beautiful, breath-taking, awe-inspiring. People around Pier Village, my apartment complex, spoke of the rainbow as some kind of miracle. Maybe it was. Or, it might have been nothing but a reflection of the sun's light being refracted through the prism of the clouds. To me, it was a symbol of hope, which included buying a new cane and moving on with my life. To express my feelings, I wrote a poem about The Rainbow of Hope. Whether or not the poem is fit for a college freshman class of English, it did serve to set me free from a morass of despair, signaling that natural events like rainbows can inspire us to have hope.

The Rainbow of Hope

Rainbow colors reverberate
in descending wave lengths,
red to purple, blood to wine.
The rainbow's arch,
embraces the sea's expanse
glowing in prismatic beauty.
I reflect on the meaning
of the rainbow, as
my eyes are transfixed,
and a smile grows
on my face.
My sadness is transformed
to a feeling of hope,
a promise of love,
shining in space.
1. From <u>Love and Hope by the Sea</u>, Tony Tripodi,
    i Universe Press, New York, 2008.

Choosing A Second Cane

Choosing a second cane wasn't exactly like getting married a second time, but there were some similarities. My first cane and I were inexperienced, and it was difficult to accommodate to each other. Shopping for the second cane was more deliberate, akin to being more thoughtful in remarrying.

I was hopeful I could find a cane that would continue to ease my pain. Yet, more aware of myself as a cane walker, I was curious as to how I was perceived.

I began my quest for a new cane at Walgreen's pharmacy in New Jersey. There weren't any canes for sale, but a pharmacist informed me about a nearby store that specialized in canes. There were an assortment of canes made of wood or metal. Although more expensive, the canes appeared to be sturdier with more character then my vanished cane.

I finally settled on a cane that I liked. It was a royal walking cane made from an imported wood of a light brown color. The tip at the bottom was surrounded by rubber. Beneath the handle, somewhat shaped like a bird of paradise, were two rings, two inches apart, that circled the cane.

The cane felt good to hold. I also discovered that it was accommodating to my human whims. I could use it to lean on, to push buttons on elevators, to ward off stray animals, to stop a dropped piece of paper from blowing away, and so forth. I felt this cane could help me walk, reduce my pain, and even enhance my appearance.

I realized the cane user's appearance depends on the type of cane used. Those who wield metallic ones appear, in general, to be like recovering hospital patients. In contrast, those who use good looking canes act as if they are well-dressed adventurers on the world scene. Could it be true that "canes make the man," in a similar way to "clothes make the man"? Whereas hospital cane bearers reek of immediate need for patient care, ornate cane users symbolize a need to be dapper, dressed for the occasion of cane wielding in modern day society.

Sadly, although I felt more accepting of the second cane and was prepared to discern differences among cane users, I continued to think about the negative consequences of cane bearing. We cane users are often perceived as older and more immobile than we actually are. Our desire is to be treated with dignity and respect. It is most certainly not our wish to be pitied.

I, as did many others, mourned for a well known horse, Barbero. He broke his legs in a race and had to be euthanized. Barbero's death inspired questions such as this. Could horses live longer if they used artificial means of transportation—canes, walkers, wheel chairs, trailers? Would humans in some kind of fascistic state be euthanized for not being able to walk or run?

Of course, it's easy to scoff at ideas such as these. They may be far fetched for some, but perfectly reasonable to others who adhere to the dictum, "survival of the fittest." Realistic or not these fantasies are entertained by myself as well as other cane walkers.

Our fantasies can be humorous and may help to relieve us of daily anxieties in the cane world. In addition, we can reduce some of the anxieties we experience by increasing our understanding of people's perceptions about canes and their users.

Cane Perceptions

Perceptions of cane users can vary by age and the type of cane employed. With respect to age I think of several groups: the very young,, young adults, middle age, and old age.

The very young span the years from toddlers to teenagers. Toddlers with canes, walkers, or wheel chairs appear to be afflicted with genetic diseases, or have been in serious accidents. I perceive them with sorrow and empathy. They are in the early stages of life, and don't have coping experiences that can help them adapt to their circumstances. Those youngsters need the loving care, tender and tough, of parents and/or guardians.

Many ailments of teenagers are due to accidents. Hopefully, those patients will soon be rid of their canes. Crutches and canes made of metal are used as walking aids for them.

Young adults are viewed with hope for their recovery and adaptation. If their injuries are due to athletic competition (e.g. broken bones), they are likely to be viewed as courageous, as athletic heroes. They recover and are able to discard their canes and crutches. In contrast, toddlers and teenagers may find accidents, and even diseases, difficult to deal with; e.g., they may be teased, and yet pitied, by their friends.

Obviously, middle age is at the cross roads between youth and old age. Middle aged persons are more likely to respond favorably and quickly to operations and rehabilitation than the elderly. If they need canes, they'll use them. However, their canes will be discarded as soon as it is convenient.

I'm in the old age category. I met some elderly persons who had hip and knee replacements. To a person, they indicated their recovery was lengthy; and they were grateful for the love and care they received from families and friends.

Elderly persons, more than younger people, are subject to those illnesses that lead to death: heart attacks, pneumonia, cancer, etc. Hence, they tend to be fearful of operations, hospitals, and nursing homes. Perhaps, not all of the elderly populations think of death when undergoing routine operations for broken bones, joint replacement and the like. However, I sometimes think of death when those operations occur. Not in the sense of suicide, but more concentrated on quasi-rational thoughts. What is death? Is it painful? How often does it occur due to the negligence of medical personnel such as doctors, nurses, pharmacists?

Our perceptions are also influenced by the types of canes employed: metallic or wooden. Those who use metallic canes are often temporarily cane persons, while those with wooden canes appear to be older. For older persons cane use is more permanent and perhaps, a precursor to the use of wheel chairs.

In my limited experience I have not observed people who use canes as an accessory to their wardrobe. Centuries ago it was common for gentlemen of the leisure classes to carry canes. Not for assistance in walking, but as a calling card.

There are many ways to describe canes, particularly with respect to their construction, physical attributes (length, weight, etc.), and the types of material from which they are made. However, none of these characteristics indicate how to perceive other cane walkers and myself. It is the psychology of the cane user that is important to me.

So, how do I perceive myself? As I described earlier, I struggled to use a cane. When I carried a cane, I thought of myself as older and helpless. Yet, I fought against those thoughts and tried to be as independent as possible. Over time, as I became used to the idea of a cane and the perception that most people want to help, I relaxed and accepted being somewhat more dependant on others. Why not? I reasoned if people want to help, I should try to make them feel good for wanting to come to my assistance. In other words, by accepting their help, I was also helping them. It may be a perverse, narcissistic point of view; nevertheless, it has been a helpful way for me to perceive others.

Rather than standing up in a bus when someone offered their seat, I sat down and thanked them. When I dropped the cane, I more readily accepted someone picking it up. At the same time, I didn't want, for example, family members doing everything for me. Somehow, being too dependent engendered feelings of helplessness. I tried to find a balance between independence and dependence. It was physically impossible for me to be extremely independent. On the other hand, too much dependence made me feel depressed and utterly useless.

As one can discern, these psychological machinations helped me to be more accepting of interactions with others. Rather than thinking of cane interactions as dark and somber, I began to see what was amusing and engaging in the human spirit.

Accordingly, what follows in Part Two are perceptions and brief vignettes about my interactions with people. Acknowledging that perceptions may or may not be factual and generalizable, I discuss my perceptions of people toward me and my changing perceptions of them.

Registering My Car

It shouldn't be complicated to register a car, especially if you clearly own it. However, with leased cars, the leasing company is the owner; and registration is more difficult. In my experience car registration in New York City was frustrating and nerve-racking. It was with my first cane, the dark brown symbol of helplessness, that I set out to register my car. I thought I had all the right papers; but according to employees of the Department of Motor Vehicles (DMV), I didn't. I needed the original copy of the lease agreement, not a duplicate. I phoned the leasing company, Jaguar Credit; and I was told I could only obtain a duplicate.

Armed with new information, I returned to the New York DMV. Again, I was informed I need the original copy of the lease agreement, not a duplicate. Back to the phone! A Jaguar Credit representative said I should tell employees at New York DMV to talk to him by phone.

I went back to DMV, wondering whether I could smell a catch-22 in the air. Naturally, DMV could not talk to the leasing company representative. This circular game went on for two more trips to DMV.

With my first cane, I acted as independently as possible, showing no signs of helplessness. The upshot of that attitude was that I was surly, arguing with whichever DMV clerk happened to be waiting on me. I was clearly at my wit's end.

After several visits to the downtown DMV, I noticed an interesting phenomenon. An Asian clerk seemed to move people quickly through his line. So, it occurred to me that I should stand in the Asian's line. ON my final trip to New York DMV I did exactly that. Lo and behold, in 10 minutes the car was registered. No fuss, no muss. It was done. Maybe it's true; Asians are smarter than the rest of us. Obviously, arguing with DMV employees was to no avail. Patience was certainly a virtue, i.e. with the right clerk.

When I moved to New Jersey, I had to register the car again. I dreaded going through all the rigamarole. However, I was more prepared for the impending hassle. I had a second cane and I was more accepting of my disability. In addition, I might have been more patient.

At the New Jersey DMV I limped with the heavy plodding of a cane walker. Prepared for the worst, I thought I had all the necessary papers in order. I approached a person who was providing information to DMV customers. Aware of my concession to the cane as a helping device and of the possibility that people like to assist handicapped persons, I limped to the DMV clerk. I made sure he knew I needed help. This is what I said:

"I'm new in the state, and I want to register my car. However, I need help to do so because I am old, slow, and handicapped."

The New Jersey DMV clerk led me to another employee who helped me through the process. It was smooth sailing!

Evidently, admitting my handicap to myself and asking for help worked wonders. Of course, one might think it was simply the fact that the New Jersey office I went to was more efficient and helpful than New York DMV. I felt it was due to a perception of myself as one who asked for help from the New Jersey DMV clerks who wanted to help. In essence, it was a cane perception that led people to help me.

I continued to use the cane to reduce physical pain. However, my psychological pain due to DMV frustrations was reduced entirely. I accepted the fact I needed help, and I perceived my cane as an asset rather than as a hindrance.

The Window Washer

In my apartment complex there are a number of boutiques, restaurants, parking spaces, apartments, and a boardwalk adjacent to the Atlantic Ocean. Apartment residents and strangers are friendly and sometimes strike up conversations. One such person was washing the windows of an Atlantic book store.

I often looked through the window, early in the morning when the store wasn't open, to gaze at the titles of new books. One day the window washer, engrossed in his job saw me peering through the windows. He asked if the windows were clean enough; and, slipping into a conversational mode, observed that I used a cane. He assumed I was retired, and in a verifying manner asked whether I, in fact, was retired. I said I was.

"It must feel good," he said.

I countered with, "It has its moments."

Not wanting to end the conversation, he talked about himself: "I'm going to retire in five years, but I'll have to put up with my wife."

The window washer indicated upon retirement his wife would want him to paint the floors in their house. According to him, she didn't understand that it would require a great deal of work. Before they could be painted, the floors needed to be thoroughly sanded. To me, it sounded like she wanted to put him to work on their house to keep him busy once he retired.

"She doesn't understand anything", he lamented. He went on to say he lived with her for 20 years, but didn't know if he could stand it if he were with her all day long.

The window washer obviously took the opportunity to complain to me, a retired person bearing a cane. Moreover, he ruminated about his retirement dreams.

Since he said his wife didn't understand him although they lived together for 20 years, I suggested: "maybe it's a good thing she doesn't understand you. Maybe that's why you're still together."

Window washer looked at me in a quizzical manner, as if I had just landed from somewhere in outer space. I could have told him to do what she says, divorce, semi-retire, or not retire at all. However, I felt it was none of my business.

I iterated how clean the windows were (thereby terminating the conversation), and I wished him the best of luck on his retirement plans. Since I didn't see any books on retirement through the cleaned windows, I wasn't able to recommend a book he might read.

Slowly, it dawned on me that he didn't want to read about retirement. In Nike fashion he just wanted to do it (but in five years). I limped away with the steady beat of my cane striking the pavement. I thought I was perceived as a sounding board that heard the echo of his words; words of a window washer who wanted to do something else with someone else in another time and place.

Woman With A Broken Hip

The apartment building in which I live has long, seemingly endless hallways. In the winter, older people can take their daily walks indoors. One afternoon while walking to the elevator in my limping manner, I met an older woman walking with a cane. Although I thought of her as elderly, she turned out to be my age. A further instance of my denial, i.e., I too am elderly.

We cane bearers stopped to talk. She said she fell on her hip and broke it. That necessitated a hip replacement. She had the operation one month previously and was still in pain. She was religiously adhering to her regimen of rehabilitation, walking twice a day in the hallways.

She asked me if I had an operation. I who have dreaded an operation said, " No, but I've been thinking about it."

She blurted out:

"Don't do it. I had no choice.
I had to do it. Thank God, my daughter has been able to
stay with me.
I don't know what I would have done without her."

Her words immediately traveled to that part of my brain that reverberated, " Don't get an operation."

The woman with the broken hip definitely wanted to get rid of her cane. It was a symbol of frailty to her. She probably imagined her cane chanting in homage to Shakespeare: "Frailty, thy name is woman."

Several months later we met again in the hallway. She observed, "I see you still have your cane."

I did have my cane. The reason she remarked about it was that she was cane free and wanted me to notice. She had a smile on her face although she seemed to limp more than she had previously. Nevertheless, she was making progress, and was proud of her efforts.

What I noticed then and even one year later was that she continually limped a great deal. Her recovery apparently was slow, which jibed with the information I received from the orthopedic surgeon Dr. OPERATE LATER. Essentially, this was more information that led me to postpone a hip replacement operation.

I recently read in USA Today (I think that was the correct source) a new study indicated that older patients recovered from hip and knee replacements just as quickly as younger patients. At first I thought that was good news. Perhaps, I should have had a hip replacement. Unfortunately, I read further. I discovered the "older" group, aged 75 and older, was compared with a "younger" group, 65 to 74. It required up to one year for members of both groups to show marked improvement. I moaned,

> "Come on! Sixty five to 74 is not so young at all. Evidently
> a 74 year old man was thought of as young while a 75 year
> old man was old!"

The study certainly didn't support stories that fans of hip operations told me, i.e., that people recovered in a week from the operation.

Obviously the study was flawed by not extending the definitions of young and old to include a range of cohorts aged in the 20's, 30's,

40's, etc. In addition, other contributing factors such as other physical ailments, types of operation, etc, were not controlled.

I still see the woman who had a broken hip. She's happy that she doesn't use a cane, and her smile seems to grow when she sees that I still use a cane. However, she limps from side to side, the way I do when I don't use a cane.

The Cane Set

I was limping along in tune with my cane when I looked up and saw two other men with canes. One had a hospital-like metallic cane; the other, a walking stick that was straight as a pole. All of us were elderly with various degrees of limping. I limped the most with the steady sound of my cane going clomp, clomp, clomp. The man with the hospital cane walked faster than I. He appeared to convey the promise of soon discarding his cane, which went hippety hop, hippety hop, hippety hop. The third man's theme was that of a gentleman. He walked lightly with a tap, tap, tapping of his walking stick. He noticed the three canes, smiled, and said:

"Here we are, the cane set."

The three of us smiled – clomp, clomping, hippety hopping, and tap tapping away.

We didn't converse, but I thought of the possibility. What would members of a cane set talk about? We could initiate our own support group, the reign of canes. Or we might discuss the various types of pain we endure, having a contest to determine which one is least bothered by pain.

On an educational note we might develop some kind of publication, entitled the cane set. We could provide news about all of the cane bearers in the area and write about special tours for cane people. We might discuss themes such as the cane set does the boardwalk or surfing with the cane set.

We could also organize and report on activities: the cane set Olympics, cane set travels, and cane set concerts. The three of us might become the cane set trio with hospital cane man playing lead guitar; the stickman, the drums; and me, strumming on the base.

I imagined that hospital cane man was eagerly looking forward to discarding his cane, professing that he's as good as new. The nattiest dressed person of the cane set, the stickman, would, no doubt, continue to bear his walking stick proudly. I, in turn, would continue to struggle about the meaning of the cane and the extent to which it would be helpful in pain management.

Perhaps, all of this was an illusion; for I have not seen the other members of the cane set again. Nor have I organized a support group or other activities focused on cane bearers.

Douglas Mac Arthur, famous general in World War II, said, after he was fired by president Harry Truman, "Old soldiers never die. They just fade away."

To paraphrase that sad refrain, "Old cane bearers never die. They just fade away, tap tapping, hippety hopping, and clomp clomping."

Deanly Advice

Deans of colleges and schools travel to many national conferences. In addition to representing their universities and discussing academic policies and their professional issues, deans can have fun. They renew old acquaintances, eat at trendy restaurants, and engage in a little site sightseeing.

A former dean and professor emeritus, I appeared at a national conference on social work research with my new cane. It was an emblem of retirement as well as a symbol of leg and hip pain.

A dean of a Midwestern college saw me walking with the cane and took it upon herself to give me some advice. She had been taking care of her husband, a former dean for many years. He too walked with a cane, but advanced to a wheel chair. Evidently, if I understood correctly, he neglected to have operations that might have enabled him to continue to walk without a wheel chair.

The dean asked me, "What's the problem?"

"I have a bad leg", I responded.

A very nice, supportive, and caring person, she said I shouldn't wait to get an operation. I should submit myself to whatever surgery is available. Strangely, she didn't pursue whatever facts or conditions were pertinent to my well-being. Probably pressed for time, she exclaimed that if I didn't act quickly, I could end up like her husband in a wheel chair. Perhaps, she was projecting a dislike of her husband's condition; for it appeared that she had to work very hard to take care of him, bringing him to conferences, and so forth. Having giving me her advice, she hurried to whatever appointment she had.

I was somewhat dismayed by her medical advice, and I wondered whether I too might wind up in a wheel chair. If so, I didn't think I would bother anyone since I was living alone. I would have liked to learn more about her husbands' progression to a wheel chair; for I might have been able to compare my situation to his.

Almost immediately after the dean departed, I met a former colleague who was a professor at a western university. He walked with crutches, and had been doing so since he was stricken with polio as a young boy. Having experienced pain in my leg, it occurred to me that he might have been beset by much more pain than I.

My former colleague told me he suffered a great deal of pain at the conference, not due to dreadfully boring meetings, but to his own physical maladies. Over the years I never thought of the pain he endured, but I did on that day. It was my own pain that made me more sensitive to his. He told me he was always in pain. That led me to realize that I could have been in even more pain than I was.

The brief encounter with my former colleague helped me to understand there are relative degrees of pain, and my situation wasn't necessarily so bad. That realization also enabled me to dilute the advice from the dean. I really didn't need to get an operation right away. Maybe a cane, along with medication, would be sufficient for managing my pain?

Cane Man's Son Gives Advice

My son is always full of advice, exotic and luxurious. He's a non-litigating lawyer, a vice president of business and legal affairs for MTV international networks. Combining skills of corporate, international, and entertainment law, he deals with lawyers and business persons from a number of countries, especially Asia.

As sons are inclined to do, he often assumed the role of acting as my father. For instance, he taught me to spend money, enjoy fine food, and to travel. Perhaps that originated from a world wide track meet of Jewish adolescents, the Macabi games, in which he ran the 1,500 and 3,000 meter races.

The track meet was in Toronto, Canada; and my son was intimidated by the athletes who came from many different countries. He didn't do as well as he could have in the 1,500 meter race, and he felt terrible. He didn't want to run in the 3,000 meter race.

Learning from my son (when he acted as my father), I said I would treat him to the most expensive Italian dinner in Toronto if he would run the next day (encouraging him to eat a great dinner and not to give up). We had an extremely enjoyable dinner, and he felt better. The next day he competed in the 3,000 meter race and performed relatively well. Who said bribes don't work?

Focusing on the subject at hand, i.e., my aches and pains, what advice could I expect? He said that if I didn't get a hip operation right away, my condition would get worse. I replied that an orthopedic surgeon who was an expert on those types of operations suggested I didn't need to hurry to be operated on.

My son, the lawyer, immediately becoming an expert on orthopedics, informed me that the medical expert, Dr. OPERATE LATER, was wrong. Nevertheless, standing my ground, I wasn't convinced I needed an operation at that time.

Having learned that he shouldn't give up so easily, he came up with a grand idea several weeks later. Possibly influenced by his interest in Asian countries, he noted it is possible to obtain inexpensive hip operations in Thailand (or was it Sri Lanka?) and be treated royally while recovering in a tropical paradise. A combination of an exotic solution with practical considerations.

The lawyer soon became aware of my stubbornness, la testa di Calabria (The Calabrian temperament.), a trait exhibited in turn by his son, my grandson. Although my son taught me how to spend money more lavishly than I ordinarily would have, I couldn't see myself leaving my fate to foreign doctors whom I trusted even less than American doctors.

After that encounter, my son desisted from arguing about why I should subject myself to a hip operation. However, every two to three weeks he'd ask: "How's your hip? When will you get an operation?"

Secretly, I tried to imagine what it would be like recovering from an operation, resting on a lounge chair, drinking Mai Tai after Mai Tai, or maybe some other exotic drink, while basking in the sun. That fantasy was overturned when I read about the devastating Tsunamis in Asia. All I needed was a tidal wave, submerging myself in the sea, especially during the monsoon season. After all, one could lose his cane in that kind of weather!

Cane Man And His Sister

With respect to a possible hip operation, my sister didn't give me any advice at all. She listened to my fears and anxieties about operations; and whether or not she agreed with me, she respected my negative opinions about doctors. The fact of the matter was that the medical profession kept my sister alive and kicking with various operations and medications. Obviously, she had much more sophistication about healthcare and medicine than I.

I once told her I was listed in Marquis' Who's Who in Medicine and Health Care. She said in a shocked manner: "What are you doing in there? You don't know anything about that!"

I agreed with her, saying I didn't deserve to be in there, but I was. And, like Forest Gump, that's all I had to say about that.

Instead of telling me what to do, she said that if I wanted to have an operation she'd take care of me until I was rehabilitated. My 86 year old sister who is a loving parent and grandparent to her progeny in California simply offered to help. I was touched, but felt it would realistically have been very difficult for her to have the responsibility to assist me.

It was clear that I couldn't argue with her desire to help. It was an expression of love. All I could do was to be grateful and move on in the struggle with pain and my cane.

Riding The Bus

In New York City I frequently rode the bus. To safely do so I had to learn how to travel with my cane. The psychology of cane use played an important part in my adaptation. By psychology I don't mean heavy thoughts like those that Cain had against Abel or that my anthropomorphic cane had against the bus. I'm referring to the attitude I had towards myself and my cane.

When I first used a cane, I was self conscious and didn't want anyone to pity me because I was old and crippled. If the bus driver said:

"Move back in the bus," I moved back in the bus.

Whatever was said, I regarded it as a command. I jumped and promptly obeyed. Probably, if the driver had said,

"Sit on the floor,"

I would have sat on the floor.

I refused seats offered to me by passengers who were seated. It was usually older and frail women who offered me their seats. So you probably have some idea as to how old and frail I must have looked. Teenagers as well as men of all ages averted looking at me; and, of course, they didn't offer their seats. I too avoided looking at them. I felt I had to act just like any other robust passenger. Nevertheless, it was often difficult; for the bus driver was determined to ensure the bus would suddenly stop, jerk, and traverse its way down 5th Avenue.

Standing passengers bumped into each other while the driver, eager to complete his route and oblivious of the welfare of passengers, drove as if it were a deadly mission.

As I became used to handling a cane, especially my second cane which had a royal handle, I turned in to a more assertive person (some might say an old codger). After all, my cane had character, and I was the gentleman who had possession of it. With that attitude change, if someone offered their seat on the bus, I graciously accepted it, smiled, and sat down. If people sitting down were younger than I and not lame, I stared at them, luring them into a seat offering.

When I got on and off the bus, I would tell the driver I was slow and needed more time. Surprisingly, drivers became courteous and helpful. It was magical!

I showed that I needed help and was humble in accepting it. The typically snotty bus drivers acted benevolently (of course, the bus drivers might have thought I was the one who was snotty and cantankerous). It was an experience similar to the one I had when registering my car. People were friendly when they spotted my cane and my limp and were especially helpful if I humbly asked for their assistance.

As my self-attitude changed from that of a crotchety old man to that of a lame person who needed help, people were more responsive. And, this even occurred on crowded buses where everyone seemed to be in a great rush. As a matter of fact, it happened in that same New York City where, as reported in the New York Daily News, people were in such a hurry they rushed by a dying patient lying on a floor in the lobby of a hospital.

At The Airport

I fly several times a year, usually to a conference or to see relatives. It is no secret there are many frustrations in flying: delayed flights for the flimsiest reasons, long security lines, jostling for storage space, and so forth. I have always tried to arrive at airports early, to be among the first in line. With a leg affliction, limping, and my cane, I have slowed down considerably. Now I need more time to change flights and to go from one terminal to another.

When I first used a cane, I was reluctant to accept help. I had to show (more to myself than to others) I was like everyone else; I didn't need extra privileges.

This was exemplified in the boarding for one flight. It was announced that anyone needing extra time could board earlier. I ignored the call. When my row was announced, and I boarded, a flight attendant said,

"You could have boarded earlier."

I told her, "I was all right. I didn't need any help."

However, I thought it might have been a good idea. On the next flight, I again didn't board early.

The third time was a charm. I did board early and it definitely made traveling easier. This, in fact, led me to demand early boarding on subsequent flights. On one flight, first class and frequent fliers were allowed to board first. I asked if I could board, and to my chagrin, I was told I couldn't. I walked away in a huff, waiting for my row to be called. One minute later, a flight attendant came to me, apologized, and said I could board right after the first class and frequent fliers did. I accepted what felt like special treatment.

Changing planes and traveling from one terminal to another was a different matter. I typically walked, noticing there were many bus-type cars for assisting passengers. I thought I would be asked if I wanted a ride. However, I was asked only after I had already arrived at my destination. In my experience, the farther away I was from my destination, the less likely was it that the airport chauffeurs (clearly a euphemism) would ask if I needed assistance. As I limped along, I saw chauffeurs talking with each other by their parked cars. They seemed to be having a good time, laughing and trading stories. I gazed at them, but they turned away. In retrospect, I should have been more vocal in expressing my desires.

I learned that most airport personnel were very helpful. However, they can't read minds; so they could only help if asked. Of course, my reasoning was fallacious. I thought that if I limped slowly (which I had to do anyway) and wore a pained expression on my face, I would be asked if I needed help. On the other hand, the chauffeurs might have thought they could read my mind; and it was clear I didn't need any assistance.

When I go to airports now, I seek all the help I can get. I don't act like I'm independent and have the capacity to fly faster than a speeding bullet, like superman, from one terminal to another. I have accepted the fact that I am slower, and it is more comfortable to accept the aid of others.

A Secondary Cane Gain

Psychologists consider secondary gains as extra benefits that patients receive when they are ill and/or are cared for by others. And, secondary cane gains can be thought of as unplanned benefits received by cane bearers, such as myself.

An example of a secondary cane gain occurred after a football game my son, an assistant professor at Florida State University, and I attended.

Before the game, we drove to the Coliseum, a venue for the Michigan Club. We were guests of another Florida State professor, my close friend, and her father for a luncheon there.

After lunch we made our way to the stadium, a 20 minute walk from where our car was parked. We rooted for the Michigan football team, but were deeply disappointed because it was soundly beaten.

Kind of dejected, we ambled slowly to the car. A Michigan employee drove up to us in a golf cart and asked if we wanted a ride. We accepted. My son smiled and indicated the ride was a welcome relief. I held up my cane and said, "Secondary cane gain." We received an unanticipated benefit from one who noticed me limping with a cane.

Cane Man Hits The Highway

I have used my cane so often that it has become an appendage. It feels like it is I who am an appendage to the cane, rather than the cane being an appendage to me. Hence my sobriquet, the cane man.

To drive a car requires some adjustment. First, I can't drive a car with a clutch since my left leg is not up to the task. Prior to my affliction I always dragged my left foot, i.e., rode the clutch, when I drove cars without automatic transmission. Henceforth, I simultaneously did a favor for myself and to clutch-operated cars by only driving cars with automatic transmissions.

Second, I had to re-learn how to get into the driver's seat. The seats are low in my x-type jaguar. I have to hold onto the roof with my left hand, balance myself with my right hand when I plop into the seat, and slowly guide my left leg into driving position.

Since I became an appendage to the cane, I had to learn how to walk with it, lean on it, and hold it while pumping gas. Moving from New York to New Jersey was fortunate. For some reason, gas station attendants pump gas for customers in New Jersey. That obviously was an easy adjustment to make.

It has been very interesting to drive on the New Jersey turnpike, especially stopping at restaurants. Limping along, I noticed many Hispanic and African American teenagers. To my pleasant surprise, teenagers noticed my cane and immediately became helpful by holding the restaurant doors for me to enter. Contrary to whatever stereotypes I might have had about minority groups and teenagers, I discovered they were respectful of my affliction as well as my age. In contrast, white teenagers didn't go out of their way to acknowledge my existence or to offer help.

Perhaps, the minority teenagers recognized me as one of them. I was a minority person in the sense that I was a cane user, and there were few cane people who stopped that day at the turnpike restaurants. In addition, I am a dark-complected Italian American and have often been mistaken as Hispanic, Indian, Middle-Eastern, or whatever group designation was in vogue.

Amazing at it seems, I discovered unity and a common bond among minorities in the turnpike restaurant. It was frequented by travelers in New Jersey where people stopped for snacks, beverages, and bathroom time. I walked away from the restaurant with a more rapid gait and less of a limp then usual.

The Value Of A Cane

It was reported in the New York Daily News (August 20, 2008, p. 10) that an 85 year old woman who lived in a Crown Heights Building was mugged from behind and robbed in the elevator. A surveillance camera showed her being choked by a 36 year old hoodlum on parole. Not only did he rob her of $900 in cash. He also took her cane.

Pictures of the event were published in the newspaper, and it inspired a middle-aged New York man to help restore her sense of dignity and independence. He did this by purchasing a cane and giving it to the woman's niece, who in turn presented the new cane to her hospitalized aunt.

The niece reported her aunt was extremely distraught about the incident, but she broke out in a big smile when she received the cane. It was her first smile since the assault, and the receipt of the cane did seem to restore some of her dignity.

The story struck a note of disgust in New Yorkers. Stealing money was one thing, but robbing an elderly woman of her cane was appalling. Obviously the value of a cane included much more than its financial cost. Perhaps, the value of the cane might have been more meaningful to the hoodlum if he only stole the cane?

I'm sure canes, walkers, and wheel chairs were also valued by the 29th Bomb Group of the U.S. Army Air Force from WWII. According to USA Today (Sept.8,2008, p.3A), veterans of the Bomb Group had their last reunion visiting the World War II memorial in Washington, D.C. Those veterans were genuine heroes, but their reunion was bittersweet; for it was a farewell reunion, the 13th since the end of World War II. Their numbers rapidly dwindled. Due to age, the 80's and the 90's and their infirmities, it had become too difficult to travel.

The quality of life for those veterans undoubtedly has been enhanced by the use of walkers, canes, and wheel chairs. I know, for me, the value of a cane is inestimable. I certainly would not want anyone to steal my cane!

A Cane Nightmare

I woke up at 3:00 A.M. one morning, went to the bathroom, and drank Gatorade. The previous evening I ate a piece of sharp cheddar cheese and drank two glasses of cabernet sauvignon from Paso Robles, California. It may not be generally true, but it seemed that my late snack (or was it the wine?) led to a nightmare. And, a ringing headache later in the morning.

I dreamt I was in Berkeley, California. I parked my car at someone's house and was told by a father of one of my son's friends to put toys in the car. Dismayed, I wandered off looking for toys. Somehow I appeared in a movie theater, and it dawned on me as I left the movie that I lost my cane. I walked to several stores, asking people where I could buy a cane. Suddenly, amazed that I could run, I ran to several stores, searching for a cane. After quite a bit of running, I was back at my car, chagrined because I found no toys and no longer had a cane.

Subsequently, I became very annoyed. An unidentified woman called me an a—hole. I wondered who gave her the right to reduce my body to one piece of anatomy that was empty, like the hole in a donut. I thought of derogatory four letter words for the woman, but woke up flustered.

I suppose a psychoanalyst could have fun trying to explain and piece together the fragments of my nightmare. It surely was not amusing. I blew my nose and took an aspirin, and my headache soon disappeared.

Yet, although I'm neither a psychoanalyst nor a rocket scientist, I noted my conflicts in the dream.

I used to love the feeling of freedom while running, but in the dream I seemed to be running away from something. With my dependence on a cane and my inability to run, except in my dream, I wanted to get rid of the cane. By discarding the cane I hoped, as if by magic, I would regain my former athletic skills. To complicate the dream analysis further, running after I lost my cane appeared to symbolize running away from having a hip replacement.

I have no idea as to what toys represented. Perhaps, putting them in a car was for their potential use at some destination, like a beach. I had recently purchased a beach ball and a shovel for my four year old grandson. Moreover, one day across the street from my apartment, my son and grandson ran on the beach in a joyful, carefree manner.

As for the woman who called me an a—hole, she may represent what my deceased father might have said. Or more simply, it might have been my recognition that she was right.

My dreams are usually fragmented with a seemingly unconnected series of events. The nightmare which included distorted memories and hidden anxieties may seem far fetched; however I, didn't make it up. I just dreamt it.

I had not thought of it before I had this nightmare, but it is possible there are two uses for my cane: to manage pain and to prevent me from having nightmares. If only I could program my unconscious thoughts to know that I have a cane, even when I dream!

An Older Cane Man

In my apartment building there are mostly young people in their 20's and 30's, with a scattering of middle aged and elderly persons. I'm in the elderly group although I have been told I look 10 years younger than I actually am. This illusion is most likely due to my skin which is bronzed and relatively smooth.

One day I noticed a short man, probably in his 80's who was walking to the elevator with his wife. She held his left arm while he used his right arm to tap the floor lightly with his cane—tap, tap, tapping in cadence to a military march in slow time. He wore ear plugs, and I thought it might have been due to hardness of hearing. However, who am I to say? He might have been, avoiding all stereotypes, listening to hard rock. When he saw me, he said, "Hello young fellow," as he smiled with a knowing twinkle in his eyes.

For some weird reason, I was immediately irked. Who was he to happily greet me anyway? There was no good reason for me to be riled. Yet, my imagination got the best of me; and I began to think he was boasting. He has lived longer than I. He is with his wife, so he has someone who makes him feel needed. And, he uses his cane in a post-operative kind of way, like a gentleman who survived his ordeals of pain, enabling him to happily tap, tap, tap along.

Obviously, my mood was due to my inadequacies and the perception there was an older man cane walking much better than I.

Chastising myself, I thought I shouldn't be so critical of others whose intentions were most likely good. Hence, I immediately suppressed the encounter.

About a month later, he approached me as I waited for the elevator on the fourth floor of my apartment building. It turned out we were neighbors. As if he were carrying on from our previous meeting he again said,

"Hello young fellow."

I said to myself maybe he has Alzheimer's syndrome, or he doesn't remember very well. Answering my thoughts, he asked whether I heard him. I indicated I did, as he allowed me to enter the elevator first. We rode to the lobby in silence; but his eyes were twinkling, and he said,

"Have a nice day."

Obviously, my theory that he had Alzheimer's syndrome was for naught. Maybe it was I who had problems with memory and memory loss.

On our third encounter, he repeated his greeting,

"Hello, young fellow."

I didn't reply,

"Hello, old cane man."

It was because he actually might have been younger than I. Or, in an imaginary vein, he might have been some kind of android who in all kinds of weather and at all times of any day was programmed to utter,

"Hello, young fellow."

Laughing at myself, I thought in one sense all of us are programmed to give daily greetings: have a nice day; have a good one; etc. Maybe it's the elevator that induces us to speak as if we are programmed. Some androids even smile, and those smiles are much more pleasant than our inane salutations. But I've come to like the old cane man. When his eyes twinkle, a smile grows on his face, and he says,

"Hello, young fellow."

With my cane I go clump, clump, clumping along. And, the old cane man happily taps away.

I'm Trying To Avoid That

A middle-aged man saw me limping with my cane. He was walking with his wife and responded to her query as to whether or not he should purchase a cane.

"I'm trying to avoid that", he said.

He was limping like me; yet, he was adamant about not wanting to use a cane. I didn't have a conversation with him, but I imagined how he was feeling. Perhaps, he was beginning to go through the same struggles I have had. Purchasing and using a cane might represent his succumbing to old age and the persistence of pain. Moreover avoiding the cane could symbolize a continuation of youth. Instead of lamenting, "Oh to be young again", he might have been thinking,

"Damn, I am still young. I don't need a stupid cane!"

A cane can elicit the fear of old age and the certainty of death. These somber thoughts are for those of us who live with a great deal of pain, which can be managed somewhat by a cane. For the healthy ones with little pain, a cane can be viewed positively. A cane can represent a symbol of power and pride, an emblem of strength. Gentleman, shepherds, hikers, and the University of Miami football fans love their CANES.

Gender Bias In The Cane World

I have often wondered whether I, a member of the cane world, am perceived differently by men and women. Although I have not attempted to conduct a study, my impression is there are differences between sexes when they relate to cane men. This is especially the case with respect to holding doors and allowing cane men to exit elevators.

The following anecdotes provide some food for thought about gender bias. The first episode took place on an elevator. Three middle aged women were in an elevator as it stopped on my floor. I entered and rode to the ground floor with them. Thinking like a gentlemen, I said to the ladies, "After you."

The good women refused to leave, insisting that I go first. There was a momentary gridlock in the elevator. No one budged. Finally, after being out stared, I departed, limping along in my usual clomp, clomp, clomping manner.

The second anecdote was a bit strange. I was walking to my car which was in the parking lot of the Long Branch library and police station. About 50 feet from my car a woman was walking toward her car. We weren't in each others' paths. Nevertheless, she maneuvered herself so she was in my path and she suddenly stopped, waiting for me to cross her path. She told me to go ahead. I innocently said that it wasn't necessary for her to wait. In an action bordering on defiance, she stood in front of me, insisting I go first. I, in turn, insisted that she keep walking to her car. She did; but as she walked away, she looked at me as if I were a little daffy since I refused her unnecessary assistance.

It occurred to me that in my experience women of all ages have gone out of their way to be helpful. However, they seemed to make sure I was aware of their honorable intentions.

In contrast, males, behaved differently particularly along racial lines. Minority males, similar to my experience in New Jersey turnpike restaurants, held doors open, greeted me, and beckoned me to go first in leaving elevators. White males were sometimes helpful but were often silent, giving a head nod in greeting. Some were completely oblivious to their surroundings. Overall, when males offered help, they were not insistent that I receive it.

More than likely these are biased observations based on skewed samples of men and women. I don't really know if there is gender bias in perceiving cane men. It may be that cane men are the biased ones in their perceptions. I am truly grateful for the help that was offered. However, in retrospect, I wish that others could have recognized my desire to be somewhat independent and to observe, even if it is not fashionable nowadays, that I rather liked being gentlemanly, allowing women and children to leave elevators first while I slowly go clomp, clomp, clomping along.

Cane Stages

As the story of my cane has evolved, I have come to recognize these stages of adaptation: stubborn independence, shaky ambivalence, greedy dependence, and realistic balance. These stages are in no way scientifically derived. They are overlapping, but they do describe my adaptation to a cane.

The first stage occurred when I bought my first cane. I had to get used to the idea of handling the cane and to what the cane might symbolize. Paying lip service to the idea that a cane is one way to manage pain, I was reluctant to accept help. As I previously indicated, I refused seats that people offered while I stood in a New York City bus. I wanted to show them I was independent. I could stand just as well as they could. Hence, I stood despite the fact it was painful. Obviously, I was struggling about accepting help from others. I was stubbornly independent.

I entered the second stage of pain adaptation when I saw the advantage of using a cane. The cane definitely reduced pressure on my sore leg and hip. However, I was ambivalent about accepting help. Sometimes on a bus I would accept a seat offered to me. Other times, I would stubbornly refuse. Often I wasn't sure as to whether I would accept any assistance. I had mixed feelings about my cane, and it was difficult to believe that people really wanted to be helpful. I oscillated between independence, not needing help, and dependence, accepting whatever help was given. I was in the stage of shaky ambivalence.

In the third stage I asked for and accepted help. I began to see the advantage of accepting assistance, regardless of whether I needed it. On a city bus, I would ask for assistance from the driver or from other passengers. At the airports I would go to the head of the line for boarding. In other words I was greedily dependent. I took advantage of my disability to obtain help from whoever wanted to give it.

I am currently trying to achieve the final stage of cane adaptation: a realistic balance. This means that I should feel it's all right to ask for help, especially when I need it. Yet, in this stage I need to do things for myself when I am physically and mentally able to do so. For example, I can carry packages in my left hand while manipulating the cane with my right hand. Moreover, I'm able to drive unassisted. Obviously, if I pressed people to drive for me, I would be retrogressing to the previous stage of greedy dependence.

Whether or not I eventually have a hip replacement, I don't envision the possibility that I'll be cane free. My cane has, indeed, become a necessary appendage.

In conclusion, I have related the story of my adaptation to a cane. The next time you see someone with a cane, you might wonder what the cane means to him or her; and what it has meant to me. If you listen carefully, you will hear me clomp, clomp, clomping along, and then tap, tap, tapping away as I fade from your view.

Notes

Notes

Notes

Notes

Notes

Notes

Notes

Notes

Notes

Notes

Notes

Notes

Notes